PRANIC HEALING

A Beginner's 5-Step Quick Start Guide on How to Get Started, With an Overview on its Health Benefits

Felicity Paulman

mindplusfood

DISCLAIMER

By reading this disclaimer, you are accepting the terms of the disclaimer in full. If you disagree with this disclaimer, please do not read the guide.

All of the content within this guide is provided for informational and educational purposes only, and should not be accepted as independent medical or other professional advice. The author is not a doctor, physician, nurse, mental health provider, or registered nutritionist/dietician. Therefore, using and reading this guide does not establish any form of a physician-patient relationship.

Always consult with a physician or another qualified health provider with any issues or questions you might have regarding any sort of medical condition. Do not ever disregard any qualified professional medical advice or delay seeking that advice because of anything you have read in this guide. The information in this guide is not intended to be any sort of medical advice and should not be used in lieu of any medical advice by a licensed and qualified medical professional.

The information in this guide has been compiled from a variety of known sources. However, the author cannot attest to or guarantee the accuracy of each source and thus should not be held liable for any errors or omissions.

You acknowledge that the publisher of this guide will not be held liable for any loss or damage of any kind incurred as a result of this guide or the reliance on any information provided within this guide. You acknowledge and agree that you assume all risk and responsibility for any action you undertake in response to the information in this guide.

Using this guide does not guarantee any particular result (e.g.,

CONTENTS

INTRODUCTION

I t is easy for us to take the energy we have available for granted as we go about our day-to-day lives. We get out of bed in the morning and immediately get to work, but during this time, we don't give much thought to the significant part that energy plays in our lives. But what if we were unable to maintain our energy levels? How would we even make it?

A major drop in quality of life would result for many of us if we were unable to maintain our current level of energy. We would experience fatigue constantly and, as a result, would probably be less productive at work or school. There's a possibility that getting out of bed in the morning will be a struggle for both of us. And if our energy levels were low for a lengthy period, we were more likely to suffer major health issues.

All facets of life require energy in some form or another. It's what keeps us alive and enables us to move, breathe, and think. It's what keeps us going whether we're putting in a lot of effort at work or when we're competing in a sport. And this is what contributes to our overall sense of well-being and good health.

When our energy reserves are depleted, though, everything becomes more challenging. We can suffer feelings of lethargy and exhaustion, and we could even have physical discomforts like headaches or stomach aches. A severe loss of energy can, in some people, result in clinical depression as well as other serious disorders. Stress, poor diet, and inadequate sleep are just three of the many factors that can deplete our energy levels.

What if, on the other hand, I told you that there was a method to increase your levels of energy without having to rely on sugar or caffeine? That there existed a technique that could rid your body of unhealthy energy and promote healing at the same time? However, there is, and it is a practice known as pranic healing.

In this beginner's guide, we'll tackle the following subtopics about pranic healing:
- What is prana?
- What is pranic healing?
- History of pranic healing
- The 3 levels of pranic healing
- How does pranic healing work?
- The 4 steps of pranic healing
- Techniques incorporated with pranic healing
- The benefits of pranic healing
- Advantages of pranic healing
- Pranic healing for specific conditions
- Differences between pranic healing and Reiki
- Risks of pranic healing
- A potential 5-step guide on how to do pranic healing on your own.
- Side effects of pranic healing

If you're interested in this holistic technique of healing, keep reading until the end.

WHAT IS PRANA?

There is a good chance that you are familiar with the term "prana," but you may be unsure of its precise meaning. The term "life force" or "energy" can be derived from the Sanskrit word "prana," which means both of these things. In yoga, prana is frequently synonymous with the term "breath." However, prana is not only the air that we breathe; it encompasses so much more. It is the energy that gives all living things their life and keeps them going.

In yoga, prana consists of the following five elements: space, air, fire, water, and earth. Each component is representative of a distinct facet of our everyday existence. For instance, space is symbolic of enlargement and liberty, but the earth is representative of rooting oneself and constancy.

One way to think of the five elements is as being in a state of perpetual motion or transformation. For instance, when you take a deep breath in, you are attracting the air (prana) from everywhere around you and bringing it into your body. When you inhale, the air element in your lungs expands, and then when you exhale, it contracts. In this sense, prana is continuously circulating through us; all we need to do is be conscious of its presence to tap into its potency.

WHAT IS PRANIC HEALING?

P ranic healing is an ancient kind of energy treatment that purifies and heals the body via the utilization of a life force, also known as prana. This practice was developed in India. It is a straightforward method that anybody is capable of learning, and once mastered, it can be put to use to cure a wide range of conditions related to one's health.

Pranic healing operates under the premise that all forms of life may be reduced to energy and that sickness results from an obstruction in the natural flow of this life force energy. It is a risk-free and efficient method for enhancing your health and well-being without requiring the use of pharmaceuticals or invasive surgical procedures. This therapeutic method is a non-invasive treatment that may be used to cure a wide range of health problems, including stress, anxiety, exhaustion, headaches, and even chronic diseases. The technique was developed in ancient China and has been utilized for thousands of years.

The fact that pranic healing is a method of self-healing is one of its many attractive features. This indicates that you will be able to learn how to administer it on your own to address your health issues. Pranic healing can also be combined with other types of treatment, such as Western medicine or acupuncture, to get the desired therapeutic effect.

HISTORY OF PRANIC HEALING

P ranic Healing is an effective method of energy healing that has been practiced by practitioners all over the world to lessen the effects of suffering and increase the likelihood of full recovery. Master Choa Kok Sui, who was born into a family with a history in yoga, meditation, and spirituality, developed this method out of a strong desire to find answers to life's most important issues. His family had a background in yoga, meditation, and spirituality.

After many years of study and investigation, he came up with the concept of Pranic Healing as a means of making these teachings not only approachable but also firmly based on scientific evidence.

Pranic Healing is being practiced and taught in schools and other healthcare settings throughout the world, including hospitals and other medical facilities. The fact that millions of patients have been successfully treated using this approach is evidence that it is an effective treatment modality.

Even though Master Choa Kok Sui died in 2007, his legacy will go on as long as some continue to study and practice Pranic Healing under his direction. Because of its capacity to alleviate pain and bring about healing on several levels—including the physical, mental, emotional, and spiritual—this method has evolved into a vital instrument for people who are looking for a way to achieve well-being and completeness.

THE 3 LEVELS OF PRANIC HEALING

Pranic Healing is an innovative and adaptable method of energy healing that is predicated on the idea that your body possesses an energetic blueprint that is responsible for regulating all elements of your health, including your mental as well as your physical well-being.

Basic level: The first level of Pranic Healing is often considered the basis of this practice since it places a strong emphasis on the fundamental ideas that underlie this method of healing. At this basic level, you will learn how to correct imbalances from the chakras and energy channels in your body to create balance and well-being throughout your entire being.

Advanced level: Once you have a firm grasp on the fundamentals of Pranic Healing, you are ready to go on to more advanced procedures, which will enable you to zero in on certain regions of your body that are suffering from malfunction or sickness. You may, for instance, target an autoimmune ailment or disease using advanced Pranic Healing methods, such as chronic fatigue syndrome or cancer.

Working with energy blockages in the meridians and nadis,

which are pathways inside the subtle body, is another significant emphasis at this intermediate level. In particular, these blocks have been connected to a range of various diseases, and they can be removed by Pranic Healing procedures such as coughing and sweeping.

Psychotherapy: Last but not least, prana, which in Sanskrit psychology refers to the "vital energy," is utilized by those who practice Pranic Healing to the highest degree possible. This strategy involves working directly with the mind to address psychological concerns such as anxiety, depression, challenges related to stress management, and other emotional difficulties such as obsessive-compulsive behavior (OCD).

The overall goal of prana psychotherapeutic techniques is not only to assist in the resolution of particular health issues but also to improve overall well-being. This is accomplished by assisting individuals in thinking more positively and feeling more emotionally balanced overall, which enables them to lead healthier lives that are filled with an improved quality of life across all dimensions.

Despite the differences between these levels, anybody may learn to employ Pranic Healing to enhance their health, alleviate the symptoms of disease or injury, and increase general well-being. Pranic Healing provides the skills and strategies necessary to produce actual results, regardless of whether you are interested in learning about this powerful approach for yourself or assisting others to enjoy improved bodily and mental health.

HOW DOES PRANIC
HEALING WORK?

T he concept of the body being surrounded by an unseen
energy field known as the aura is the foundation of the
practice of pranic healing. Seven levels make up the aura,
and each one correlates to a particular chakra, which may be
thought of as an energy center. Chakras are the energy centers in
the body that are responsible for regulating the passage of prana,
or life force, throughout the body. One's physical health, mental
health, or emotional health can suffer if one or more of the
chakras become blocked or out of balance.

Pranic healing is accomplished by directing the flow of vital life
force energy toward parts of the body that are most in need of it by
the use of one's hands. This procedure contributes to the removal
of blockages and imbalances, which in turn allows the body to
recover itself.

Pranic healers do not touch their patients in any way, in contrast
to the practice of conventional forms of healing, which entail
direct contact between the healer and the patient. Instead, they
merely place their hands over the bodies of their patients and
concentrate on directing the energy to the parts of the body that
require it the most. Pranic healers can assist restore balance to

our internal systems and promote healing on both a physical and emotional level by accessing our pranic fields in this manner.

THE 4-STEPS OF PRANIC HEALING

Pranic healers use three simple steps to promote healing and balance in their patients:

1. Scanning: The first thing that has to be done is to look over the patient's body with the healer's hands to see if there are any regions of energy blockage or imbalance. The sections of the aura that are strong and healthy will look brighter and clearer, in contrast to the parts of the aura that are congested with negative energy and will appear darker or more opaque than other parts of the aura.

2. Cleansing: As soon as the healer has determined which parts of the patient's aura have energy blockages, they can begin clearing these obstructions by employing their hands as a type of energetic "vacuum cleaner." During this stage, the practitioner will remove any surplus negative energy from the patient's body before releasing it into the surrounding environment.

3. Replenishing: In the last phase of pranic healing, the patient's energy stores are replenished with fresh, positive energy that originates from the environment rather than from within the body. This helps to bring back equilibrium and harmony, and it also adds to the development of general health and well-being.

4. Stabilizing: After the energy of the patient has been revived and restored, the healer will employ specific procedures to assist in maintaining this new positive energy within the body of the patient. This stage is designed to assist avoid other imbalances from forming and to keep the patient on the path toward long-term recovery and well-being.

Even though the precise mechanisms by which this energy therapy works are not yet fully understood, many practitioners believe that it can promote healing by helping to clear energetic blockages and imbalances in the body. This is even though the exact mechanisms by which this energy therapy works are not yet fully understood. Pranic healers can assist us to access our innate healing skills and restore health and vigor to all aspects of our lives by activating our inner life force and enabling it to flow freely throughout the body.

However, this is not something that can only be done by pranic healers. Pranic healing is something that may be learned by everyone and used in everyday life. Continue reading to find out more about the stages that are involved in pranic healing, as well as some basic ways that you can use to include this powerful healing approach into your routine for self-care.

TECHNIQUES INCORPORATED WITH PRANIC HEALING

P ranic healing is a practice that requires both a precise set of skills and an intuitive awareness of the energy body to be effective. Learning to scan and detect obstacles or imbalances in the flow of energy throughout the physical and subtle bodies is an important part of this practice, and one of the most significant components of this practice is learning to do so.

However, once a barrier or imbalance has been found, practitioners have access to a wide variety of diverse approaches that they may utilize to reestablish balance and facilitate healing. A healer could apply any one or more of the following techniques, depending on the location of the block or imbalance as well as the degree of it:

Pranayama: Pranayama, often known as breath control, is an essential practice that is frequently utilized in pranic treatment. To channel one's energy and fix whatever imbalances it may have, this technique requires one to concentrate their thoughts on their breathing. In particular, pranayama is beneficial for reducing stress and enhancing overall mental clarity. It entails a variety of breathing activities, such as regulated breathing, deep breathing, breathing via alternative nostrils, and so on.

Visualization exercises: These exercises consist of mentally seeing colors and light as they surround parts of the body that require healing. This helps to trigger the right energy response. We can send healing energy to the places of our bodies that require it the most by imagining these colors and surrounding those areas with light, which will finally bring our bodies back into equilibrium.

Chanting and sound vibration: One can direct tremendous life force energy into regions of weakness or pain in the body by intoning certain words or vibrating specific sounds. Pranic healers can identify blockages and manipulate prana via the use of this method, which enables prana to flow unimpeded throughout the entire system. Pranic healers can produce measurable results at the physical level by concentrating on the power of vibration and resonance rather than the power of direct energy transfer.

Meditation: A straightforward meditation practice is typically employed as one of the methods in pranic therapy sessions. This entails bringing the mind to a state of peace by concentrating on one's breathing while simultaneously letting go of any ideas or anxieties that come to mind.

Pranic healing practitioners can harness bigger quantities of energy and deliver more effective care to their patients when they learn to still the mind and achieve a more tranquil state of being. The practice of meditation helps to improve overall health and well-being by lowering levels of stress and improving mental clarity and peace of mind. This is another benefit of the meditation technique.

Mindfulness practices: Mindfulness practices are an important part of pranic healing, and they're employed as one of the essential approaches to support optimum recovery. These activities are intended to assist in redirecting our attention away from the problems and distractions of daily life so that we may instead tune into our bodies and pay attention to any signals that may come through. Through practices that help us relax and concentrate, we may heighten our awareness of the processes taking place inside of us, which, in turn, enables us to handle issues with our health in a more effective manner.

Pranic healing is an effective kind of alternative medicine that has been practiced for many decades to channel vital life force energy and reestablish equilibrium throughout the body. You, too, can start incorporating pranic healing into your daily routine and start reaping all of the advantages it has to offer as soon as you have a grasp of the procedures that are involved in this practice.

THE BENEFITS OF PRANIC HEALING

There are numerous advantages to engaging in pranic healing, regardless of whether you are seeking relief from a particular health condition, wanting to enhance your general quality of life or both. Pranic healing may help you in all of these ways. The following are some of the most significant advantages that may be gained through engaging in this potent energy therapy:

Boosted immunity: It has been demonstrated that prana healing may strengthen one's immune system and provide protection against the disease since it promotes the body's innate capacity for self-healing. Pranic healing has the potential to assist enhance an individual's resistance to infection. This is accomplished by improving circulation throughout the body and stimulating the flow of new, oxygenated blood to all organs.

Mental Clarity: One of the most significant advantages of pranic healing is that it can help to cleanse one's mind, which in turn enables one to better concentrate on one's objectives and to maintain calmness in the face of adversity. Pranic Healing is an approach that tries to restore harmony to the flow of chi throughout the body by employing practices such as breathing exercises, guided meditations, and visualizations.

It is possible to acquire a more in-depth comprehension of what is occurring inside oneself if one brings attention to the many components that make up their existence. Because of this heightened awareness, one may have improved mental clarity, enhanced decision-making ability, and enhanced potential for attaining success in all aspects of life.

Increased Vitality: Those interested in enhancing their health and vigor can take advantage of the many benefits provided by pranic healing. This one-of-a-kind method of energy therapy involves filling the body with rejuvenating prana to bring about an increase in the vital life force that is already present. People report feeling more powerful, more energized, and more alive when there is an abundance of prana in their systems.

Enhanced mood: In particular, the management of vital energy, which is promoted by pranic healing, contributes to an improvement in one's mood. Pranic therapy has been shown to successfully enhance good mood as well as lessen feelings of worry and tension. This is accomplished by increasing the quantity of healthy energy that is circulating through the body and clearing toxic energy blockages.

Additionally, pranic therapy can assist to improve one's internal defenses against bad emotions or ideas. This is accomplished by restoring balance and harmony to the subtle energies that are found inside the body. People who engage in pranic healing typically note that it has led to an increase in their levels of happiness and contentment compared to how they felt before they began the therapy.

Inner peace and tranquility: Pranic healing is a form of alternative medicine that focuses on working on the energy level to treat patients, to bring about beneficial changes in both the physical and mental planes of existence. Pranic healing provides a sense of inner calm and tranquility, which can lead to increased general well-being. This is perhaps one of the most significant advantages of this form of alternative medicine.

Improved sleep quality: One of the primary advantages of pranic healing is that it may result in an improvement in the quality of one's sleep. Pranic healing can assist you in falling asleep more quickly and remaining asleep for longer lengths of time. This is accomplished by eliminating any impurities or poisons that may be disrupting your natural sleep cycles, as well as clearing away any energy blocks that may be present in the body.

Balanced hormonal levels: When it comes to maintaining hormonal levels that are healthy and balanced, many individuals turn to traditional treatments such as hormone replacement therapies or pharmaceuticals that are prescribed by a doctor. Nevertheless, these therapies may be accompanied by a variety of unwelcome adverse effects, such as gastrointestinal distress, changes in mood, vertigo, and headaches.

A more effective substitute is pranic healing, a form of alternative medicine that restores the body's equilibrium via the utilization of the sun's and the earth's vital energies. Pranic healing can help restore hormonal balance without producing any negative side effects since it uses energy to speed up the body's natural healing processes.

Pranic healing works by utilizing energy to accelerate the body's natural healing processes. In addition, due to the customized nature of the treatment, it is adaptable to the particular requirements of the patient as well as their desired outcomes.

Faster recovery from illness or injury: Pranic healing is a potent and successful kind of alternative medicine that makes use of the body's energy to facilitate a speedier recovery from disease or injury. Pranic healing was developed in India in the 1970s.

Pranic healing, in contrast to other methods, which rely on external sources of power such as medications or surgery, works by strengthening the body's innate ability to mend and heal itself at the level of the cells and tissues. Pranic healing may be practiced by anybody, anywhere, at any time. Patients can recover from illnesses such as cancer or heart disease, as well as injuries brought on by accidents or those sustained during sports, more quickly as a result of this.

Prosperity and good luck: Pranic healing is a one-of-a-kind and very effective kind of energy medicine that may assist one in increasing their chances of financial success as well as good fortune. This technique entails making use of the vital energy of the body to induce healing on all levels, including the physical, emotional, mental, and spiritual ones. Pranic healing's beneficial impacts are a direct outcome of the modality's capacity to fortify and cleanse our energy systems, which, in turn, results in an enhanced capacity to bring prosperity and fulfillment into our own lives.

These are but a few of the numerous advantages that may be gained through the practice of pranic healing. This natural form of therapy can help you achieve greater physical health, mental clarity, and spiritual well-being by removing energetic blockages and promoting the flow of fresh, revitalizing energy throughout the body. This can be accomplished by clearing away energetic blockages and increasing the flow of energy.

ADVANTAGES OF PRANIC HEALING

P ranic healing is a powerful form of energy medicine that has many advantages over other healing modalities.

Pranic healing can successfully be applied to a wide range of conditions.
Pranic healing is a kind of complementary and alternative medicine that has shown promising results in the treatment of a diverse variety of diseases and conditions. Pranic healing, in contrast to many other forms of treatment, places its emphasis not on external intervention or surgical procedures, but rather on the body's innate capacity to mend itself. Because of this, it may be utilized even in the most delicate circumstances, such as those with diseases that are chronic or fatal.

Pranic healing is safe and does not have any side effects.
Pranic healing, in contrast to a great number of other forms of alternative medicine or therapies, does not come with any potentially harmful side effects or hazards. In addition to this, the focus of this mode of treatment is on enhancing the body's innate capacity to repair and rejuvenate itself.

Patients who receive pranic therapy report feeling better and healthier overall, as a result of the treatment's ability to promote the body's natural healing process. In general, it is abundantly obvious that pranic healing is a risk-free and efficient method that does not include any undesirable side effects or risk factors in any manner to enhance overall well-being.

Pranic healing is a drug-free treatment option.
Pranic healing, on the other hand, does not call for the use of any specialized tools or training, in contrast to more conventional medical treatments that rely primarily on pharmaceutical medications and intrusive procedures. Instead, what it does is provide the body with a concentrated amount of life force, which is how it functions. This energy can either be directly administered to afflicted regions of the body using a gentle touch, or it can be absorbed in the form of food and drink to restore the natural equilibrium of the body from the inside out.

Pranic healing is a simple and convenient way to receive energy healing.
Pranic healing provides a straightforward and hassle-free approach to enhancing one's health and well-being at any time and in any location, in contrast to other forms of energy healing practices, which call for the application of tools and methods that can be difficult and time-consuming to master.

Pranic healing can be practiced in place of these other forms of energy healing practices. Pranic healers can change the energy patterns inside the body by engaging in focused breathing exercises and using a gentle touch. This has the effect of removing blockages and increasing flow throughout the entire system.

Pranic healing can be done by anyone, regardless of their level of experience or training.
You may learn to channel your energies in such a way as to have a beneficial effect on the energy systems of others no matter how much experience or training you have had in the past. Because

there are numerous materials accessible to assist you in learning pranic healing procedures, anybody who has an interest in improving their health and well-being may get started right away.

Pranic healing techniques have been used for thousands of years. You may become an adept pranic healer and take your practice to the next level by devoting yourself to the practice and working on developing the abilities essential for this profession.

Pranic healing is an affordable way to receive energy healing.
Pranic healing, in contrast to traditional medicine, which can be both expensive and intrusive, centers largely on the use of energy to facilitate the body's natural ability to heal itself. Because of this, pranic healing may be learned and practiced by virtually anybody who has a fundamental understanding of how energy work operates. As a result, people looking for alternative forms of therapy will find that pranic healing is an option that is both accessible and cheap.

Pranic healing is a holistic treatment option.
The holistic practice of pranic healing, which is often referred to as energy healing, focuses on rebalancing and reestablishing connections within the body's energy system. It is possible to improve one's general health and well-being via the practice of pranic healing. This is accomplished through encouraging balance and strengthening one's immune system. This way of thinking about health provides a lot of individuals with helpful insights into how they might enhance their own lives by making dietary and lifestyle decisions that are more beneficial to them.

PRANIC HEALING FOR SPECIFIC CONDITIONS

Pranic healing is a type of energy therapy that has been practiced for hundreds of years to cure a wide range of medical issues, ranging from minor aches and pains to more severe diseases. It has been demonstrated that pranic healing is a beneficial treatment for a variety of particular illnesses, including but not limited to anxiety, depression, chronic pain, digestive difficulties, and more.

Cancer: Cancer is a dreadful illness that affects millions of people all over the world, and pranic healing is a successful treatment for the condition. This kind of treatment is effective because it targets the energy patterns that lie at the root of cancer. By doing so, it liberates the body from obstacles and enables it to cure itself.

Traditional therapies for cancer, such as chemotherapy and radiation therapy, also benefit from this therapy's assistance. According to the findings of several studies, pranic healing has the potential to assist in raising the quality of life of cancer patients by improving their physical health, mental health, and a general feeling of well-being.

Depression: Pranic healing is an effective treatment for depression because it treats both the mental and physical parts of this prevalent disorder. Pranic healing is also known as "energy healing." Pranic treatment is effective on a physical level because it helps to increase the flow of life energy, also known as prana, through the body.

This enhanced flow can assist to normalize the autonomic nervous system, which in turn can help to reduce some of the symptoms of depression, such as having a low mood and having trouble sleeping. Pranic therapy can also treat the mental part of depression by inducing positive thinking patterns and heightening self-awareness. Pranic healing is a form of alternative medicine.

Anxiety: Pranic healing practitioners can assist clients in alleviating the symptoms of anxiety and improving their general feeling of well-being by removing "blockages" in their energy fields. In addition, this approach is very beneficial for those who do not react favorably to standard therapeutic methods, such as taking medicine or participating in psychotherapy. If you deal with anxiety and are seeking a natural solution to ease your symptoms, pranic healing may be the option that is most suited to meet your needs.

Stress: It has been known for a very long time that pranic healing is an effective method for lowering levels of stress and enhancing emotions of relaxation and overall well-being. This method of energy treatment is non-invasive and works by focusing on the subtle energies that surround the body. This has the effect of increasing general vigor as well as mood and mental clarity.

There is mounting evidence to suggest that pranic healing can be especially helpful in addressing the effects of chronic stress. This method involves working directly on the chakra system to assist in clearing blockages within the energy grid of the body. This, in turn, makes it possible to restore the normal flow of prana inside the body.

Chronic pain: Pranic healing has the potential to be very helpful for people who suffer from chronic pain since it can assist to calm inflamed and irritated tissue, alleviate stiffness and tension, and lessen pain sensitivity. In addition, this treatment is effective because it takes a holistic approach, meaning that it takes into account the individual's mind as well as physical health. Therefore, for those people who are seeking an alternative method to reduce chronic pain, pranic healing may be worth looking into.

Infertility: Practitioners can assist in the restoration of balance and vigor to the reproductive system by removing obstructions from the energy fields and restoring the natural flow of prana, also known as the life force. And since it targets the underlying energy reasons of infertility directly, pranic therapy can often be more effective than traditional medical approaches in treating the condition.

Because of this, many couples who have had difficulty conceiving a child turn to this method as a last resort after they feel like they have exhausted all of their other choices. Pranic healing has the potential to be a useful tool for reaching your objectives and constructing a happy and healthy family, regardless of the method of conception you want to pursue (i.e., naturally or through assisted reproductive technology).

Digestive issues: Pranic healing can assist to ease symptoms such as bloating, cramps, and diarrhea by concentrating on increasing healthy energy flow throughout the body. Pranic healing is a form of alternative medicine. In addition, therapy of this kind is quite effective in alleviating chronic health issues such as Crohn's disease and irritable bowel syndrome.

Heart disease: Heart disease, which can be brought on by a variety of different things, is one of the conditions for which pranic treatment is sought most frequently. In the treatment of heart disease, two of the most important aspects of pranic healing are increasing the amount of oxygen that is taken into the body and reducing inflammation.

This is often done by a mix of particular breathing exercises and dietary choices, such as those that are high in omega-3 fatty acids and antioxidants. Some foods that are high in these nutrients include: In addition, certain medical professionals may recommend particular mental exercises or methods of stress management to enhance patients' cardiovascular health.

Diabetes: It has been demonstrated that pranic healing can assist in lowering levels of stress, which is known to be a significant component in the development and progression of diabetes. This method of treatment is effective because it restores equilibrium in the patient's emotional state, enhances nutritional intake, and enhances blood circulation. Practitioners can construct individualized treatment regimens that are catered to the specific requirements of each patient when they combine a variety of holistic methods with energy work.

Without just depending on medicine, it is feasible to effectively control diabetes and keep healthy blood sugar levels by making use of these specific treatments as opposed to relying solely on medication. The use of medicine is no longer necessary for the majority of diabetic patients who have undergone pranic healing to cure their condition.

Pranic healing may assist you in accomplishing your health-related goals and leading a lifestyle that is both healthy and balanced if it is practiced with the appropriate mix of techniques and methods. This sort of holistic treatment can improve both your physical and mental well-being for the better, which is beneficial whether you are searching for a way to get relief from chronic pain or are trying to conceive naturally.

DIFFERENCES BETWEEN PRANIC HEALING AND REIKI

Both Reiki and Pranic Healing are examples of popular energy based healing practices that have been around for many years and have a long history of use. There are some parallels between the two techniques, but there are also several important distinctions to be made between them.

- In pranic healing, the practitioner channels energy from the sun into the patient, whereas in Reiki, the practitioner channels energy from a higher spiritual source, such as the universe.
- Pranic healing is thought to increase energy levels and promote healing, whereas Reiki is believed to provide relaxation and stress alleviation. Pranic healing can also be used.
- Pranic healers are not required to have any special training or certification before they may practice, in contrast to those who practice Reiki, which requires a particular level of attunement before they can work.
- Pranic healing makes use of light touch as an integral part

of the treatment process, in contrast to Reiki, which does not involve the use of touch to transmit energy.

- Pranic Healing leans more largely on sweeping methods and directing energy into specific problem areas, whereas Reiki places its primary emphasis on channeling energy through the hands.
- Pranic healers are required to actively extract energy from their surroundings, but Reiki practitioners do not need an external source of energy for their practice to be effective.

In the end, despite these distinctions, Reiki and Pranic Healing are equally effective methods for fostering physical, mental, and emotional well-being in their practitioners. It is up to you to decide whether the calm flow of Reiki or the more concentrated approach of Pranic Healing better suits your needs.

RISKS OF PRANIC HEALING

Even though proponents of this technique believe that prana healing may assist to alleviate pain, enhance energy, and cure sickness, there are various hazards linked with prana healing.

Drug interactions and allergic responses during recovery.
The possibility of adverse interactions between pranic practices and medically prescribed drugs is one of the most significant sources of worry. For instance, certain pranic practices have the potential to change the way a person's body metabolizes particular pharmaceuticals, which might result in these prescriptions being more or less effective.

People who are allergic to or hypersensitive to particular herbal ingredients that are utilized in pranic therapy are also at an increased risk of experiencing adverse effects from receiving the treatment. Before beginning pranic healing, one must thus ensure that they are informed of all of the potential dangers involved.

Limited research.
Pranic healing is a practice that involves extracting healing energy from one's surroundings to treat a variety of health issues and

illnesses. Even though there has been a rise in interest in this method over the past several years, there has been very little study done to determine whether or not pranic healing is successful in treating the ailments in question.

Before deciding to use pranic healing as a kind of treatment, it is essential to take into consideration several significant dangers, given that the potential advantages of this approach are not yet fully understood.

In the first place, there is always the possibility that only relying on pranic healing might cause a delay in the identification and appropriate treatment of potentially life-threatening or otherwise significant medical illnesses.

When a patient already struggles with symptoms of anxiety or depression, the likelihood of them finding solace in the belief that they have discovered an alternative treatment method rather than seeking assistance from sources that are more traditionally used increases, which can make this risk more severe.

In addition, patients may be unable to identify specific triggers for symptoms or side effects that could point to an underlying issue rather than simply being caused by their condition itself if they do not have the input and guidance of a trained medical professional. This can increase the likelihood that the patient will experience further complications as a result of their condition.

When considering whether or not to include pranic healing in your strategy for obtaining optimal health, it is crucial to take into account both the proven benefits and the potential drawbacks associated with the practice.

It is essential to have a conversation with a trained medical practitioner before receiving any therapy including pranic healing. Doing so will help lower the hazards involved with the practice. In the end, the decision about whether or not an individual is willing to put himself in harm's way to potentially reap the advantages of pranic healing rests solely within their control.

A POTENTIAL 5-STEP GUIDE ON HOW TO DO PRANIC HEALING

Here's a potential five-step guide to help you get started with pranic healing:

Step 1. Grounding:

The process of grounding oneself is the first stage in prana healing. This is an important step since it creates the foundation for all subsequent types of healing and energy-based treatments. Before commencing the grounding technique, it is vital to clear your mind and body of any distractions or obstacles that may be present.

This may be accomplished by meditating or using some other form of deep breathing. This can be performed by engaging in exercises that focus on deep breathing, practicing practices that are connected with meditation, or by envisioning energy flowing freely throughout one's body. These are just a few examples.

Step 2. Scanning/Tuning In:

After you have released all of the tension and stress that was stored in your mind and body, you are now prepared for the next stage, which is to scan the energy field surrounding you to locate regions of the body that may require healing. You may accomplish this by imagining energy flowing through the body, or you can just tune in to your intuition to learn where potential barriers are located in the body.

Step 3. Applying Prana:
The third step consists of applying prana, which is also known as the energy of the life force, to the regions where there is a blockage. It is possible to accomplish this objective and assist in improving the flow of prana by making use of various visualization techniques, focusing on specific chakras, employing essential oils, herbs, crystals, or any of a variety of other natural healing approaches. All of these methods are excellent ways to accomplish this goal.

Step 4. Releasing:
When you have finished scanning or tuning in, the next step is to release any blocks or bad energy that have been found throughout this process. You may accomplish this by imagining these energies leaving your body, or you can release the energy by participating in physical activities such as exercise or yoga. Both of these methods are effective.

Step 5. Integrating:
The final phase in pranic healing is to integrate any positive shifts that may have happened as a result of the previous steps. You can conclude this step of the process by engaging in more meditation or by keeping a diary in which you reflect on your experience with pranic healing. Additionally, to preserve any beneficial changes that may have happened as a consequence of pranic healing, it is essential to keep up a healthy diet and way of life. Pranic healing may be found here.

After the procedure, you will most likely experience a sense of relaxation, centeredness, and connection with both your body and your environment. There is a significant possibility that you might benefit in a variety of ways by engaging in the practice of pranic healing, regardless of whether you decide to make it an ongoing component of your medical care or only experiment with it as a stand-alone modality.

However, before beginning, it is essential to have an open dialogue with a qualified medical expert and keep in mind the potential dangers that may be involved. You may gain the numerous advantages of pranic healing while simultaneously lowering your likelihood of encountering unpleasant side effects or other unfavorable impacts, provided that you employ the appropriate strategy.

SIDE EFFECTS OF PRANIC HEALING

P ranic healing is an alternative therapy that involves the use of energy to heal the body. While there can be many benefits to this practice, there are also some potential risks and side effects that should be considered.

Increased feelings of stress or anxiety: One possible side effect of pranic healing is increased feelings of stress or anxiety. This may occur due to the intense visualization exercises involved in this process, or simply as a result of heightened sensations and awareness during treatment.

Increased energy levels and feelings of fatigue: Another possible side effect is increased energy levels and feelings of fatigue. This may occur as a result of the body releasing built-up tension and blockages, leaving you feeling both invigorated and exhausted afterward.

Changes in the balance of hormones: Alterations in the levels of hormones or other chemical compounds in the body are another potential consequence of receiving pranic healing in some instances. This may disrupt the normal healing process that your body is attempting to go through and may cause you to have side effects such as changes in appetite, mood fluctuations, or digestive problems.

Pranic healing may be associated with a small number of potentially adverse effects; however, they are not severe and may be readily avoided by adopting an incremental and attentive strategy when engaging in this practice.

CONCLUSION

Your physical health and mental well-being can both benefit in a variety of ways by undergoing pranic healing, which is a very potent and efficient kind of energy therapy. This holistic technique makes use of the remarkable curative potential of vital life energy, also known as prana, to assist restore balance, boosting vigor, and creating a sense of serenity and tranquility.

Pranic healing can help alleviate chronic pain, improve the quality of sleep, boost mental clarity, and strengthen immunity against illness by clearing blockages or stagnation in your subtle energetic bodies and chakras. Pranic healing is practiced by clearing blockages or stagnation in your subtle energetic bodies and chakras. This transformational practice is incredibly helpful for stress reduction and relaxation, enabling you to naturally lower levels of tension and concern in your day-to-day life. In addition, this practice is extremely good for stress release and relaxation.

It is essential to keep in mind that although pranic healing is becoming more well-known as a potent alternative to traditional forms of care, this practice should still be utilized in concert with other techniques to provide oneself with adequate self-care.

Pranic healing may help us enhance our health and well-being by tapping into the innate healing capacity of our bodies. However, depending solely on pranic healing is not enough to achieve good physical and mental health on its own. We need to make sure that we receive plenty of exercise and eat a balanced diet in addition to engaging in this practice if we want to get the full advantages of it.

In addition, it is essential to schedule daily time for pranic healing. We may do this by enrolling in a class at a nearby studio that lasts for one hour or by listening to guided audio recordings to learn how to channel energy and remove blockages from our bodies when we have free time. We may start reaping the numerous advantages of pranic healing, including improved health, more pleasure, and an overall sense of well-being, by engaging in these straightforward activities.

FAQ ABOUT PRANIC HEALING

1. Can you explain what pranic healing is?
Pranic Healing is an energy medicine method that dates back more than 5,000 years and is considered an ancient kind of healing. It is predicated on the idea that the human body is made up of energy, and that this energy may be channeled to cure the physical self.

2. What is the process of Pranic Healing?
Pranic Healing is effective because it makes use of the body's energy to restore health. The practitioner will use their hands to channel healing energy into the body of the patient, which will assist to support the natural healing process that occurs inside the body.

3. Can you tell me about the advantages of pranic healing?
Pranic Healing is associated with several health advantages, some of which include the alleviation of stress, the promotion of better sleep, an increase in one's energy level, and a fortification of one's immune system. In addition, Pranic Healing is a successful treatment for a wide variety of illnesses affecting both the physical and emotional health of patients.

4. Who may take advantage of receiving pranic healing?
Pranic Healing is a non-invasive and gentle form of treatment that is suitable for individuals of all ages and can be of help to everyone who receives it.

5. How long does a session of Pranic Healing typically last?
A Pranic Healing session usually lasts for thirty to sixty minutes on average. However, to the requirements of the patient, sessions may be either shorter or longer in duration.

6. How many appointments do I need to schedule?
The number of sessions that are necessary will change based on the ailment that is being treated as well as the individual's reaction to the treatment. In general, the majority of people will require anything from three to ten sessions to see meaningful changes in their health.

7. What kinds of things might I anticipate happening during a session?
During a session, you will either recline in a plush chair or lie down on a table designed specifically for massage. In several predetermined locations on your body, the practitioner will put their hands either above or softly touching your body. During the session, you can experience several different feelings, such as warmth, tingling, or pulsating sensations.

8. Are there any potential adverse reactions?
The practice of Pranic Healing is a kind of treatment that is risk-free and has no known adverse effects. However, when their bodies acclimate to the increased energy flow throughout the session, some individuals may suffer momentary discomfort either during or after the session. In most cases, this soreness is not severe and it passes very fast.

REFERENCES AND HELPFUL LINKS

"5 Most Effective Energy Healing Techniques and How They Work." The Times of India. The Economic Times - The Times of India, https://timesofindia.indiatimes.com/life-style/health-fitness/home-remedies/5-most-effective-energy-healing-techniques-and-how-they-work/articleshow/70698807.cms. Accessed 25 Nov. 2022.

"7 Easy Steps To Do Pranic Healing Meditation." STYLECRAZE, 18 Aug. 2014, https://www.stylecraze.com/articles/easy-steps-to-do-pranic-healing-meditation/.

"About the Founder." Light of Pranic Healing, https://lightofpranichealing.be/pranic-healing/about-the-founder/. Accessed 25 Nov. 2022.

Can Reiki and Pranic Healing Be Dangerous? https://isha.sadhguru.org/us/en/wisdom/article/reiki-pranic-healing-dangerous. Accessed 25 Nov. 2022.

Home - Pranic Healing Foundation of the Philippines. https://pranichealing.com.ph/. Accessed 25 Nov. 2022.

MD(Ayu), Dr J. V. Hebbar. "Pranic Healing – Meaning, Method, Benefits." Easy Ayurveda, 18 Feb. 2021, https://www.easyayurveda.com/2021/02/18/pranic-healing/.

Pranic Healing | The Pranic Healers. https://www.thepranichealers.com/pranic-healing. Accessed 25 Nov. 2022.

---. https://www.thepranichealers.com/pranic-healing. Accessed 25 Nov. 2022.

"What Is Pranic Healing." Pranic Healing Research Institute, https://www.pranichealingresearch.com/pranic-healing. Accessed 25 Nov. 2022.

"---." Pranic Healing Research Institute, https://www.pranichealingresearch.com/pranic-healing. Accessed 25 Nov. 2022.

What Is Pranic Healing. https://www.worldpranichealing.com/en/what-is-pranic-healing/. Accessed 25 Nov. 2022.

Printed in Great Britain
by Amazon

23106545R00030